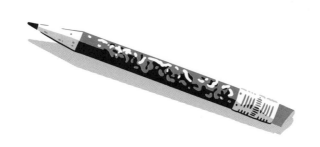

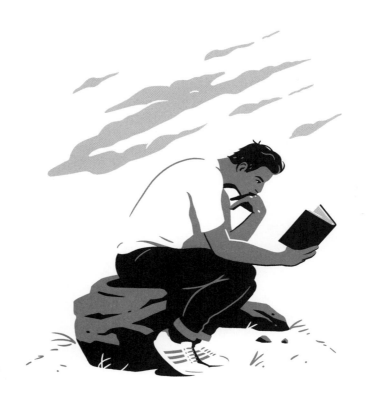

I want to concentrate

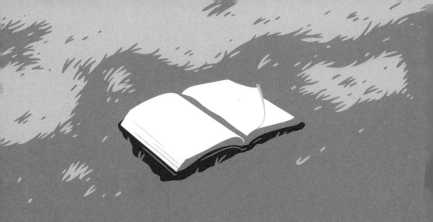

For Tony Visconti, who knows how to concentrate & with style

Other books in the *I want to...* series:

I want to sleep
I want to be calm
I want to be organised
I want to be happy
I want to be confident
I want to be creative

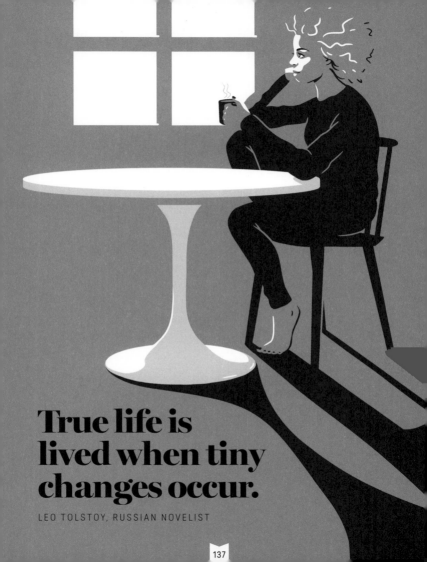

True life is lived when tiny changes occur.

LEO TOLSTOY, RUSSIAN NOVELIST

Acknowledgements

The work of so many people has contributed to my understanding of concentration, and they are all credited in the text of the book. Special thanks, though, are due to all the team at Hardie Grant with whom I've had the pleasure of working, but especially Kate Pollard, Kajal Mistry, Molly Ahuja, Eila Purvis and Rebecca Fitzsimons. Thanks, too, to Julia Murray for bringing her magic and skill to the design and illustrations.

Appendix

Further reading

Finding Flow, Mihaly Csikszentmihalyi (Basic Books, 1998)

In Praise of Slow, Carl Honoré (Orion, 2005)

Making Habits, Breaking Habits, Jeremy Dean
(Oneworld Publications, 2013)

Spark! How exercise will improve the performance of your brain, John Ratey
(Quercus, 2010)

The Art of Concentration, Harriet Griffey (Rodale, 2010)

The Artist's Way, Julia Cameron (Macmillan, 2016)

The Brain That Changes Itself, Norman Doidge (Penguin, 2008)

The Inflamed Mind, Edward Bullmore (Short Books, 2018)

The Miracle of Mindfulness, Thich Nhat Hanh (Rider, 2008)

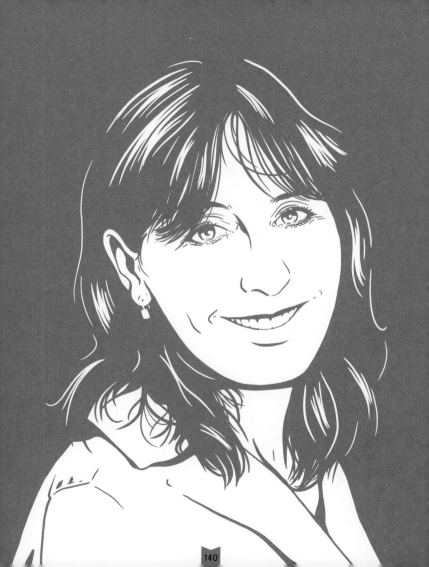

I want to concentrate

IMPROVE FOCUS AND ACHIEVE MORE

—————— BY ——————

Harriet Griffey

Hardie Grant

B O O K S

Contents

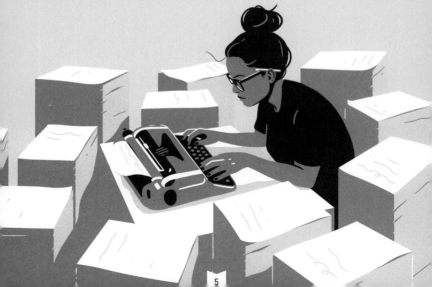

Why concentration matters

It's difficult to imagine, now, what life was like before our personal and professional lives were so constantly 'switched on' via smart phones and the other media devices that make us accessible and, crucially, so easily distractible and interruptible every second of the day. This constant fragmentation of our time has become the new normal, to which we seem to have adapted with ease, but there is a downside. Over time, it also seems that these constant interruptions and distractions have eroded our ability to concentrate effectively.

/kɒns(ə)nˈtreɪʃ(ə)n/   The action or power of focusing all one's attention.

Does it matter?

Does it matter if we don't concentrate as well as we might? Some would argue not, but increasingly we see how trying to function in this way is less efficient, more time-consuming and increasingly stressful. In turn, this erodes our concentration further and the harder we try to function in this fragmented way, the more difficult it can become. Instead of trying harder to function in this state, perhaps we should consider trying differently, and taking the steps necessary to restore some balance and learn to concentrate better.

Research carried out by Dr Glenn Wilson at London's Institute of Psychiatry found that the persistent interruptions and distractions at work had a profound effect.

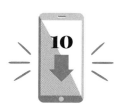

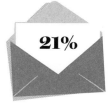

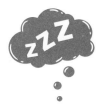

Those distracted by email and phone calls saw a 10-point fall in their IQ, twice that found in studies on the impact of smoking marijuana.

More than half of the 1,100 participants said they always responded to an email 'immediately' or as soon as possible, while 21 per cent admitted that they would interrupt a meeting to do so.

Those constantly breaking away from tasks to react to interruptions suffered similar effects on the mind as the loss of a night's sleep.

Why concentrate?

The simple answer to this is that if we concentrate better, life can actually become easier and less stressful. To do this means reflecting on what is currently getting in the way of our ability to concentrate well, and taking steps to implement the changes that can make the difference.

This may mean being more disciplined about our use of communication technologies; being more organised with our time; learning how to prioritise demands; factoring in more work life balance to allow for a more relaxed, flexible focus, which could yield better personal and professional outcomes as a result.

This may mean taking a step back from the 24/7 treadmill, allowing the time to do one thing more purposefully by creating the head space to concentrate more effectively. Once you have relearnt the skill of concentration, it becomes much easier to draw upon it when you need to really focus.

One reason so few of us achieve what we truly want is that we never direct our focus; we never concentrate our power. Most people dabble their way through life, never deciding to master anything in particular.

Anthony Robbins, American author and life coach

Better relationships

Better concentration will also help improve personal relationships. You'll be more engaged, less forgetful, more attentive to your immediate surroundings and those within them, whether this is your partner, your children or your work colleagues. It's impossible to be properly connected to someone if you are on your phone, texting, checking social media or preoccupied in some way. Everyone responds positively to good attention and, in being more attentive, you can benefit from reciprocal attention, personally and professionally.

Give whatever you are doing and whomever you are with the gift of your attention.

Jim Rohn, American entrepreneur and motivational speaker

Why concentration matters

Whether you want to reduce stress, enhance your creativity, improve your mood, have better relationships, become more consciously mindful, up your physical or mental game and, ultimately, become more productive overall, improving your concentration will be of huge benefit in all of this, whatever your age or circumstances.

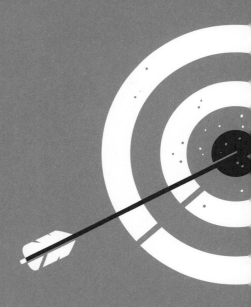

The secret to success in any human endeavour is total concentration.

KURT VONNEGUT JR., WRITER

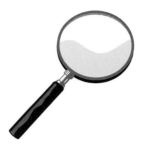

What's your concentration like?

Take this quick quiz to review how well you concentrate.

> **How much time do you spend working or thinking about work?**
  A   I only think about work during office hours.
  B   About 12–14 hours a day, I find it hard to switch off.
  C   I never stop: I pretty much think about work all the time.

> **How long does it take you to 'get into a book' that you're reading for pleasure?**
  A   No time at all – I read all the time, anywhere.
  B   I find myself re-reading the previous pages every time.
  C   Ages. Reading doesn't really hold my attention.

> **How often do you misplace personal items like your keys?**
  A   They're usually where I've left them.
  B   I can usually find them in one of several places.
  C   I'm always losing them.

> **On a train journey, how do you spend your time?**
  A I like to use the time to relax and enjoy the ride.
  B I try to catch up on some work.
  C Usually by checking social media on my phone.

> **When you cook, do you follow a recipe?**
  A If I'm cooking something for the first time, I like to get it right.
  B I get a rough idea and then put it together.
  C I don't often cook and find it irritating to follow a recipe.

> **How easily do you fall asleep at night?**
  A Within 10 minutes of putting out my light.
  B It takes me a while as I keep having to check various things before I settle.
  C I fall asleep quite quickly, but often wake in the early hours.

> **How often do you check your phone for emails or messages?**
  A I check a couple of times a day when I remember.
  B As soon as an alert goes off on my phone.
  C I constantly check my social media, even without the alerts.

> **Are you usually on time for meetings and appointments?**
  A Yes.
  B I'm usually juggling numerous things so often get delayed.
  C No, because I often forget until the last minute.

> **In a conversation, do you find it easy to listen to what's being said?**
  A Yes, I'm a good listener.
  B I'm often distracted by my own thoughts when I'm listening.
  C I tend to interrupt, even when I try not to.

> **Assembling flat-pack furniture, how easy do you find it?**
>
> **A** If you follow the instructions, it's usually quite straightforward.
>
> **B** I find it tricky to get it done as quickly as I'd like.
>
> **C** I usually get stuck halfway through and have to ask for help.

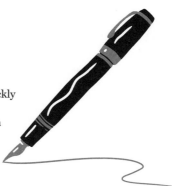

Answers

Mostly As

Generally your ability to concentrate serves you well and, if you do find yourself lost in thought, it's not usually to the detriment of what you're trying to achieve. You can increase your ability to focus by deliberately alternating between low- and high-stimulation tasks, so you don't become complacent about your levels of concentration.

Mostly Bs

You may find it helps to slow down and deliberately focus on what you're trying to do, in order to get things done more efficiently. Deliberately removing distractions while you're trying to concentrate could be a useful first step: turn everything to silent for at least 30 minutes and begin to lengthen your attention span.

Mostly Cs

If you've become so overwhelmed and frenetic through trying to do too many things at once, it will become increasingly difficult to concentrate and the stress of this may be beginning to show. You may need to take drastic steps at first to factor in new strategies that will help to support better focus, yielding better outcomes in work, rest and relationships.

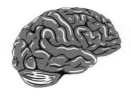

How the brain works: The science bit

At birth, our brains may be small and smooth, but almost all the brain cells – around 100 billion of them – are in place. By the age of four, the brain is around 95 per cent of adult size. At adolescence, the brain is adult-sized, if not fully mature; we now know that it takes until the mid-twenties to optimise its function. It's all those connections and neural pathways that develop in response to stimuli (continuing to do so throughout our lives) that enable the brain to perform an astonishingly wide range of functions, from the automatic blinking of an eyelid to complex abstract thought.

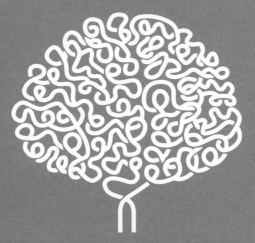

If the human brain were so simple that we could understand it, we would be so simple that we couldn't.

EMERSON M. PUGH, RESEARCH ENGINEER AND SCIENTIST

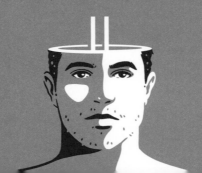

Neuroplasticity

Even if the brain no longer increases in size after adolescence, it still has lots of potential for making new connections through a process called neuroplasticity. This is as a result of new experiences or activities and, given the chance, can continue throughout life. Neuroplasticity can also make recovery possible after brain trauma or injury from strokes or accidents, to regain function or compensate for damaged areas.

NEUROPLASTICITY CAN BE HELPED BY:

- Learning new activities that link and challenge both physical and mental ability.
- Choosing activities that start relatively easily and progress, keeping you at the threshold of challenge.
- Keeping things novel and surprising to help increase focus.
- Good nutrition (page 29).
- Physical exercise (page 121).

Distraction

External and internal distractions – that is, both external stimuli like other people, traffic noise or our phones, and internal preoccupations like thought processes or mood (page 57) – need to be managed. When something is very interesting to us, we notice little else and are totally absorbed in the activity with which we are engaged. That engagement is enough to temporarily focus our attention completely.

This is much more of an automatic process in young children – we can see their total absorption in something that engages their attention – but as we become more aware of our stimulating environment, and actively seek this out, we become increasingly knowledgeable of all the things that can disrupt our concentration. This can be especially true in adolescence (page 24) with all its complex demands and as the brain begins a process of reorganisation.

Concentration is the secret of strength.

RALPH WALDO EMERSON, AMERICAN PHILOSOPHER AND POET

Using less to achieve more

It may sound counterintuitive, but you use less rather than more of your brain when you are concentrating well. That's what a study carried out by John Milton at the University of Chicago in 2006 showed. He studied the brain activity of expert golfers and compared it with that of novice golfers and, as the expert golfers concentrated on the shot, only one small area of brain activity showed up. With the novice, all sorts of activity in the brain showed up in a number of different areas. It seems that the expert golfers' ability to filter out extraneous and distracting information gave them the edge when it came to concentrating. For the novice golfers, all sorts of other irrelevant thought processes were distracting them and reducing their focus, diminishing their ability to concentrate on that shot.

This ability to focus, sometimes referred to as 'being in the zone' or 'flow' (page 85), is a good example of being in a state of extreme concentration. Those whose occupations demand high levels of focus actively work to enhance this, consciously heightening their powers of concentration to support professional excellence, from footballers to chess players.

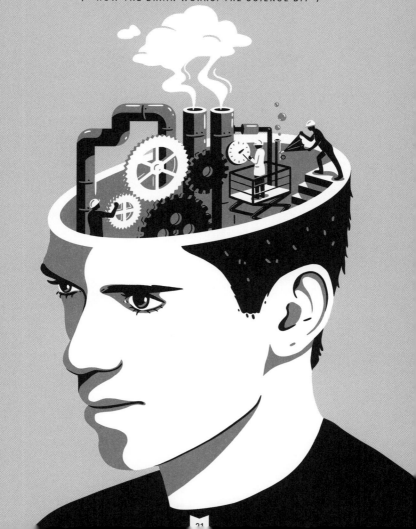

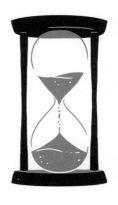

Concentration from cradle to grave

From the minute a baby takes its first breath at birth, the brain starts to react, respond and adapt to the stimuli it receives from life outside the womb. While all the brain cells were already there, all the neural pathways and the connections between them develop in response to stimuli received via the senses of sight, smell, hearing, touch and taste.

   When your survival relies on adapting to your environment and making sure that it supports you, there's already a necessity to focus and pay attention even if not consciously. So, for example, the distance at which a baby's eyes can initially focus is about 30 cm (12 in), roughly the distance to a parent's face when being safely held. This first, expressive canvas of the parental face, radiating attention, is focused on intently in return as parent and child bond. Through this first engagement, the seeds of concentration are sown.

As the world becomes more reliable, that same focus and attention once given to a parent's face begins to expand outwards. Within safe limits, all exploration is unconsciously done in pursuit of finding out how to use and manage the world, building up knowledge along the way. Watching a small child concentrate on a toy or a game, to the exclusion of all other distractions, demonstrates that this engagement is not something that has to be taught, but is there from the start.

The adolescent brain

It's worth pausing a moment to consider what's going on in the adolescent brain as it matures to adult capacity, not least because it helps in the understanding of teenagers and their sometimes erratic behaviour. Just behind the forehead is the frontal cortex of the brain, responsible for what is called 'executive function' because it's in charge of our capacity to do more than one thing at a time, plan future tasks, direct our attention and control impulsive behaviour.

During adolescence, the brain goes through a period of change where there is a shift of emphasis from the numbers of brain cells to their connections and an increase in myelin, which insulates and protects them, allowing for faster connectivity and transmission of information. In time, this will allow for better-organised behaviour and decision-making, but

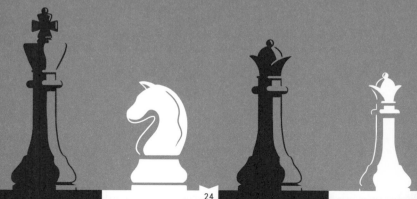

in the interim there's a period during which teenage behaviour can seem highly irrational, risky and counterproductive.

Until this processing of the grey and white matter of the brain is done, many teenagers seem to struggle with concentration (unless on a mind-numbing computer game maybe), remembering things and generally being organised ... but it will improve.

The ageing brain

Between the adolescent and the ageing brain there's a long period where if we avoid too many distractions, bad habits and are healthy, our concentration should be a reliable resource. As we live longer we have an associated risk of age-related decline in our mental powers, but even then there's good evidence that concentration needn't be impaired. And we're increasingly beginning to understand the role played by being mentally and physically active in staving off decline.

This steady and undissipated attention to one object, is a sure mark of a superior genius; as hurry, bustle, and agitation, are the never-failing symptoms of a weak and frivolous mind.

LORD CHESTERFIELD,
LETTERS TO HIS SON, 1774

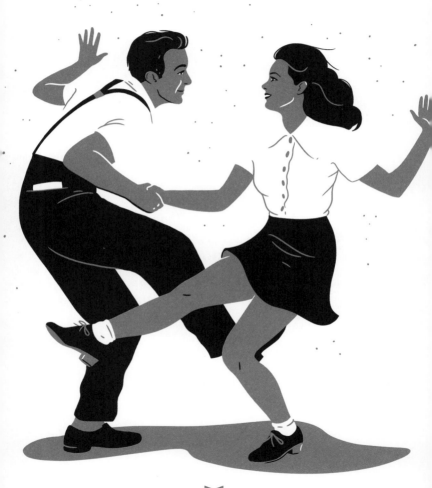

Not all activities are equal in this regard. Those that involve genuine concentration – studying a musical instrument, playing board games, reading and dancing – are associated with a lower risk of dementia. Dancing, which requires learning new moves, is both physically and mentally challenging and requires much concentration.

NORMAN DOIDGE, PSYCHIATRIST & AUTHOR OF *THE BRAIN THAT CHANGES ITSELF*

While there's inevitably some short-term memory (page 115) impairment – although this is quite different from that experienced by someone with a diagnosis of Alzheimer's disease – and a lengthening response time (our ability to retrieve information), if you remove this element of difference from standardised tests, ageing adults can perform as well as younger adults. In tests that depend on vocabulary, general information and well-practised activities, older adults show negligible age-related deterioration. And when it comes to concentration, there is no reason why this shouldn't be as good as anyone else's, all other factors being equal.

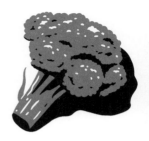

What your brain needs to concentrate

While it's helpful to reduce external distractions (page 35) to improve your concentration, it's also useful to consider what your physical brain needs to function well. It is, after all, a part of your physical body and like your other major organs, from heart to liver to gut, benefits from being taken care of.

Nutritious foods
We hear a lot about 'brain food' and the brain runs on carbohydrates, which provide the fuel for energy, as do all the operating systems of the body. This doesn't mean that it benefits from mainlining sugar, although a sugary snack can give flagging brains a bit of a (temporary) boost, but like the rest of the body the brain really benefits from good, balanced nutrition. That means enough high-grade protein from animal sources, plus a wide range of protein from vegetable sources for vegetarians, along with fruit and vegetables to ensure a good supply of vitamins and minerals, in addition to the carbohydrates.

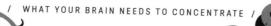

Breakfast like a king, lunch like a prince and dine like a pauper.

ANON

Low GI carbs

Choose carbohydrates with a low-glycaemic index (GI) to ensure slow-release energy and avoid excessive insulin production, which will make your blood sugar levels spike up and down. The less processed your food, the lower its glycaemic index and the better its nutrient value, so avoid refined sugars, instant or easy-cook foods, and choose oats, whole grain breads, freshly prepared or raw vegetables, high-fibre fruits, brown or basmati rice, nuts and pulses (legumes). Don't dismiss frozen or tinned vegetables out of hand, as they sometimes have a better nutrient value than those flown halfway around the world; and if you can, opt for local, seasonally available produce over the limited (and often more expensive) benefit of being organically grown.

Super foods

Some foods get dubbed 'super foods', often because they are high in antioxidants that help protect our DNA from inflammation and damage. These include berry fruits like blueberries and raspberries, tomatoes, broccoli, spinach, turmeric and black, green and white tea. Mix it up and keep exploring for lots of variety in your diet for maximum benefit to your brain.

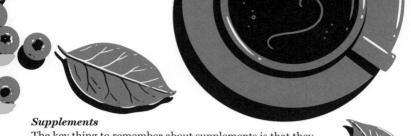

Supplements

The key thing to remember about supplements is that they should be supplementing a good diet, rather than compensating for a poor one. So before considering what supplements might be a good way to improve your concentration, look first at improving the quality of what you eat every day. An iron deficiency in particular, because iron is so important for the oxygenation of the blood, can leave you feeling both weary and brain-fogged. Make sure there are enough iron-rich foods, and the vitamin C to aid its absorption, in your diet. If unsure, check with your doctor who can arrange a quick blood test of your haemoglobin (Hb) levels.

Omega-3 essential fatty acids (EFAs)

One supplement that is sometimes recommended to improve concentration is omega-3 fatty acids EPA (eicosapentaenoic acid) and DHA (docosahexaenoic acid), available from oily fish like mackerel, herring, salmon and tuna. It seems that your grandmother was right – fish *is* good for the brain! Also, because our Westernised diets tend to be high in omega-6 fatty acids, from vegetable oils and cereal-fed animals, definitely don't supplement with these, just the omega-3s. Ideally, the balance between the two should be 1:1, whereas for many the ratio is as high as 15:1 and is thought to contribute to the high rate of modern inflammatory diseases like cancer, diabetes and heart disease.

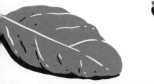
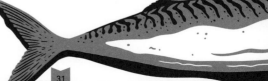

There's also thought to be a link between inflammation and mood disorders like anxiety and depression, according to recent research carried out by Edward Bullmore, Professor of Psychiatry at the University of Cambridge in the UK, so the anti-inflammatory benefits of omega-3 supplementation might be of value there as well. If you do choose to supplement with omega-3 EPA and DHA, make sure you choose a pharmaceutical-grade product with high concentrations of the active ingredient, not just a lot of fish oil. Around 1,000 mg of active ingredient (EPA) is considered a therapeutic daily dose, rather than 1,000 mg of fish oil (which may contain very little active ingredient), so be sure to check.

Hydration
You probably already know that around 60 per cent of the adult body is water, and the brain is higher, around 80 per cent. So your brain will function better when it's well hydrated. Initial symptoms of dehydration include tiredness, headaches and reduced alertness. If the condition persists, mental performance – including memory, attention and concentration – will continue to deteriorate in direct proportion to dehydration.

In 2005, the UK's Expert Group on Hydration (EGH) published a report, *Drinking in Schools*, based on research carried out at 82 secondary schools in 10 local authorities around the UK. It found that nearly half of all children were not drinking the recommended amount of 1.2 litres (40 fl oz) a day. EGH spokesman Dr Paul Stillman said, 'A huge focus has been given to children's nutritional intake, and rightly so, but we are concerned that hydration is at risk of being overlooked ... Without adequate hydration at school, a child is at risk of experiencing headaches, lack of concentration and digestive problems. This could potentially have a devastating effect on quality of study and performance, as well as adversely affecting health and general wellbeing.' As a consequence, a number of recommendations were made and implemented and teachers noticed an improvement in learning and behaviour outcomes.

Oxygen

While the brain only accounts for about 2 per cent of body weight, it uses about 20 per cent of the body's oxygen intake because of its high metabolic rate (the amount of energy used per unit of time), which is about three times as much oxygen as muscles use. It needs a good oxygen supply to convert blood glucose to energy, so without it, the brain struggles. Iron-deficiency anaemia can affect the oxygen-carrying capacity of the blood (page 31), but other factors that can cause problems to the brain's oxygen levels include high or low blood pressure, heart disease, diabetes, excessive alcohol intake and smoking.

Basically, what's good for a body's wellbeing is also good for the brain, which will, in turn, improve the ability to concentrate.

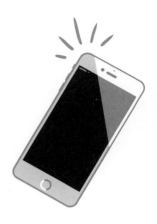

What gets in the way of concentration?

The single biggest thing that prevents us concentrating is usually external distractions. Every time you take time out from what you're doing to check your emails, for example, it takes around 15 minutes to regain your previous level of concentration afterwards.

There's a lot that's immediately under our control when we want to improve our concentration and we should be mindful of this. We can turn off our phones, email, text message and other social media alerts, along with the television or radio, while we allow ourselves to concentrate on whatever it is we want to achieve or enjoy – whether that's getting a piece of work done or watching a movie. We can create a calm, quiet environment that reduces those external distractions and allows us the possibility of concentrating better.

Don't dissipate your powers; strive to concentrate them.

GOETHE, GERMAN WRITER

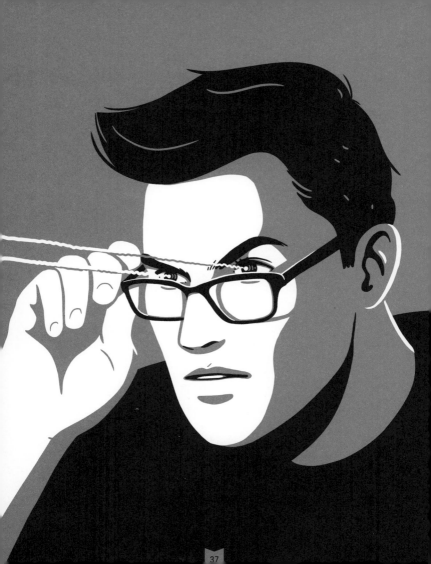

External distractions

Other external distractions may be more difficult to manage, especially if we work in open-plan offices or are exposed to traffic or building noise. While some of us have extraordinary powers of concentration, this can be more challenging to manage and take some thought. In this case, noise-cancelling headphones, sitting with your back to a window or colleagues (without offending them) or listening to music that actually aids concentration (page 112) via headphones might help. Anything that distracts you and interrupts what you are doing will impinge on your concentration, so it's worth doing what we can to reduce this.

When it comes to our external environment, it's not just noise that can make it difficult to concentrate. If we are too cold or too hot, if the lighting glares, we are hungry, thirsty or in physical discomfort, this will also distract us from concentrating well.

Continuous partial attention

Continuous partial attention – or CPA – was a phrase coined by ex-Apple and Microsoft consultant Linda Stone, who identified how, over the last 30 years, we have pushed ourselves to the extreme. By adopting an always on, anywhere, anytime, anyplace behaviour, we exist in a constant state of alertness that scans the world, but never really gives our full attention to anything. This, in turn, creates a false sense of anxious engagement, which is both stressful in the long term but also saps our ability to concentrate in the short term.

Many of us feel the 'shadow side' of CPA – overstimulation and lack of fulfilment. The latest, greatest technologies are now contributing to our feeling of being increasingly powerless. Researchers are beginning to tell us that we may actually be doing tasks more slowly and poorly.
Linda Stone, writer and consultant

Internal distractions

It's not just external distractions that can impede concentration. Internal distractions – the chattering monkey of our thoughts, worries, preoccupations – can make concentration difficult, too, as can our mood (page 57). In some ways, this is more difficult to deal with because it is not necessarily so easy to 'turn off' our thoughts or how we are feeling. However, some of those internal distractions are aggravated by external ones, so it's well worth dealing with those first, calming everything down and then seeing where that takes you.

Concentrate all your thoughts upon the work at hand. The sun's rays do not burn until brought to a focus.

ALEXANDER GRAHAM BELL, SCIENTIST

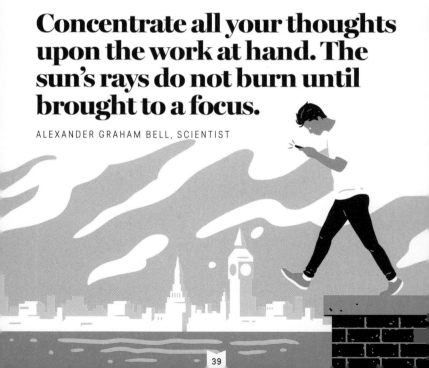

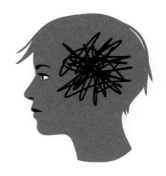

The stress of multitasking

If you want to concentrate better, give up multitasking.

It's almost as simple as that. There's some multitasking that we can easily do when one of the tasks is very routine or semi-automatic, and we take this for granted. Listening to the radio while washing up, knitting or even driving has little impact on being able to fully concentrate on what's being heard. And in some cases listening to music while we work can actually aid concentration and enjoyment as it filters out other distractions.

Multitasking is stressful

Our brain is highly adaptive and because of its neuroplasticity we can manage a variety of tasks at once, but the myth of multitasking lies in the word itself: we're not actually *multitasking* but switching rapidly between different activities and this, in the long term, reduces our productivity. In a word, multitasking wastes time, increases the possibility of errors and, what's more, it's stressful because it requires increased amounts of stress hormones cortisol and adrenaline to do. None of this matters much in the short term – these hormones are designed to support us through bursts of sudden intense activity – but in the long term this can have a negative effect. Cortisol, in particular, can knock out the feel-good hormones serotonin and dopamine in the brain, those that help us feel calm and happy, affecting our sleep and heart rate and making us feel jittery. And it's hard to concentrate when our mood is affected (page 57).

Each man is capable of doing one thing well. If he attempts several, he will fail to achieve distinction in any.

PLATO, ANCIENT GREEK PHILOSOPHER

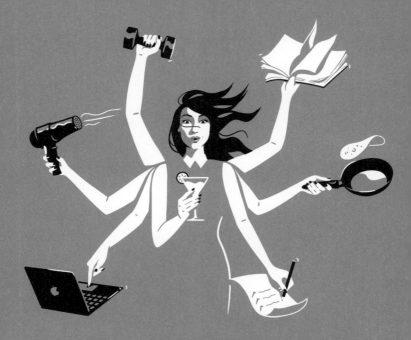

We often multitask in ways that we don't even recognise as multitasking, but it has the same effect. Every time we take a break from what we're doing to check an email or text, or Twitter feed or Instagram account, it takes 15 minutes to regain that earlier level of calm concentration that enables us to complete a task efficiently and well. This constant adaptation to interruption, and the effect of this 'continuous partial attention' (page 38), also has an impact on memory processing and the retention of information, which explains why we constantly forget things. It's not early-onset Alzheimer's disease, but overload!

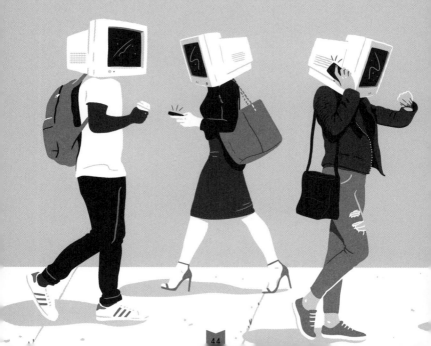

Undivided attention

We would do well to remember that a bit of undivided attention can go a long way in improving matters. So, while a proficiency in multitasking suggests that it is a good and useful skill – and women, in particular, are often praised for their ability to do many things at once – the efficiency of multitasking, except for the most inconsequential or routine of tasks, is a myth.

It's also worth remembering that the first use of the actual word 'multitask' came from a 1965 IBM report describing the capability of a computer! We are not machines and we probably need to rethink our commitment to the mythic benefits of multitasking because, as researchers have been making clear, in the long run it actually does us very few favours.

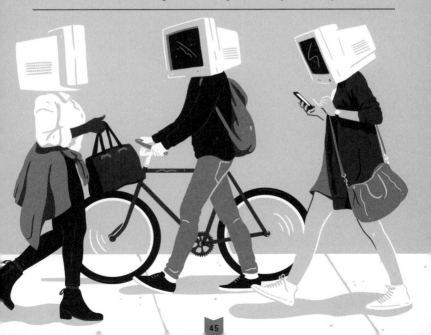

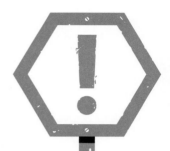

Pay attention!

We are expert in ways to sabotage our ability to pay attention: we distract ourselves, procrastinate, daydream, multitask and this becomes – and feels – normal. And as long as it feels normal, we persist, but it's worth thinking about how much easier it would be to stay on task and accomplish those things we would like to achieve, if we would only just pay attention.

WILLIAM JAMES

In 1890, doctor, psychologist and philosopher William James (brother of novelist Henry James) wrote in his book *The Principles of Psychology* about the differences between 'sensorial', 'intellectual' and 'passive' attention and, in particular, the 'grey chaotic indiscriminateness' of those incapable of paying attention. Talking about how our thoughts flowed, or not, he wrote: 'On the whole easy simple flowing predominates in it, the drift of things is with the pull of gravity, and effortless attention is the rule … But at intervals an obstruction, a set-back, a log-jam occurs, stops the current, creates an eddy, and makes things temporarily move the other way.' Today, even if our minds work in similar ways, the 'obstructions' to our ability to pay attention contribute to that 'chaotic indiscriminateness'.

Switch off to switch on

In 2018, new research from the UK's telecoms regulator Ofcom reported that, on average, people check their smart phones every 12 minutes, with 71 per cent saying they never turn their phone off and 40 per cent saying they check theirs within five minutes of waking. Just managing – switching off – your smart phone may help in switching concentration on. Both Facebook and Instagram announced they were developing new tools for their apps, to limit usage, in response to claims that excessive social media use can have a negative impact on mental health.

The ability to concentrate and use time well is everything.

Lee Iacocca, American executive

If, after any interruption, it takes up to 15 minutes to concentrate fully again, this can really cut into the time it takes to get something done effectively. It's very easy to get sucked into compulsively checking anything from Twitter to emails and then, once distracted, wasting time. Better to reduce the possibilities for this and allow your brain the benefit of better concentration.

TURN OFF:

 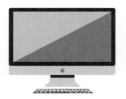 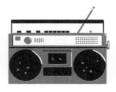

Any alert on your smart phone: calls and texts can wait.

Email alert on your computer, laptop or other device you're working on.

Unless it provides white noise, turn off any background noise like the radio or television; even then, consider turning it off.

Once you discover how much easier it is to get things done without interruptions, you will find this easier to do. Better to focus exclusively for an hour, then take a break, than muddle through for three hours, with constant interruptions, over the same thing.

The faculty of voluntarily bringing back a wandering attention, over and over again, is the very root of judgement, character, and will.

WILLIAM JAMES, PHILOSOPHER AND PSYCHOLOGIST

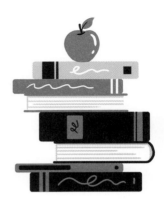

How to study – at any age

Watching small children play, their absorption in a game or activity is so complete that it is difficult to distract them. Needing to learn and remember so many new skills means there's a natural inclination to focus on one thing at a time to achieve this. We were all like that once and it's worth considering a return to it.

For anyone trying to get work done, but for students in particular, constantly switching between assignments, chatting on WhatsApp, scrolling through Reddit, googling for information, answering a text on their phone and watching the latest must-see on Netflix is just not going to help.

A study published as long ago as 2006, from research carried out by psychology professor Russell Poldrack, showed that it was difficult, if not impossible, to learn new information while distracted. 'We have to multitask in today's world, but you have to be aware of this,' he said. 'When a kid is trying to learn new concepts, new information, distraction is going to be bad, it's going to impair their ability to learn.'

Exams
Exams are predominantly a feature of young people's lives and those in full-time education, but can also occur in adult life and require considerable concentration. Preparing for exams can create a lot of anxiety, so revising well can be key – not only can effective revision reduce the stress of exams, it can also improve the results.

To be able to concentrate for a considerable time is essential to difficult achievement.

BERTRAND RUSSELL, PHILOSOPHER

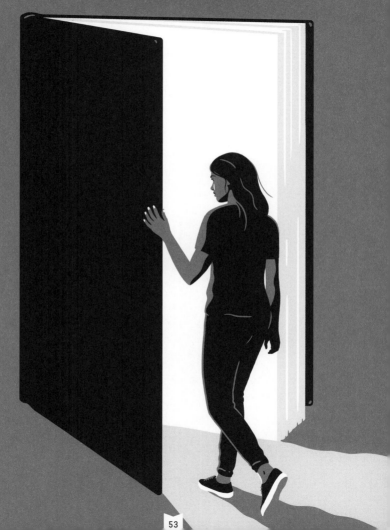

EXAM SURVIVAL GUIDE

1. Map out what needs to be done several weeks in advance and create a revision timetable with realistic daily goals leading up to the exams, allowing enough time to avoid feeling stressed too close to the actual exams.

2. Make sure that all notes, past papers, books and other sources from which to revise are available. Check in with teachers or course advisers to make sure you have everything you need before you start.

3. Utilise your own, best learning style. Auditory learners find that reading or saying things out loud, recording these and playing them back to listen to, may help things stick. Visual learners find taking notes or making diagrams a useful way to remember as they revise.

4. Allow enough uninterrupted time during a revision period to reach a point of concentration where information is actually retained and transferred from working memory into long-term memory, from where it can be retrieved when taking the actual exam. Without this process occurring, the possibility of actually remembering what has been revised is limited. This means revision periods of 20–30 minutes minimum, building on this to stay concentrated for up to 90 minutes before taking a break. If this is a new way of working, it may take time to accomplish (page 109).

5. Take time out from studying to wind down before sleep, however. The brain works best when well-slept, and chronic tiredness affects memory and exacerbates feelings of being overwhelmed.

6. Cut out distractions – all of them – during each allocated revision period. This means turning off mobile phones, instant messaging, email, Facebook and other social networking sites, and making revision a primary and exclusive focus.

7. Regular exercise in between daily revision sessions – just taking a walk, going for a run, swimming, playing football – not only helps to relieve physical and mental tension, but also increases the brain's ability to work well.

8. Eat well – the brain thrives on complex carbohydrates to keep it going, and lots of fluids to stay well hydrated, but avoid highly caffeinated drinks that claim to help concentration, as these can hype the body up and increase feelings of stress.

9. Keep a sense of perspective. Exams are a means to an end, not an end in themselves, and those who don't achieve great exam results can still go on to live happy and accomplished lives.

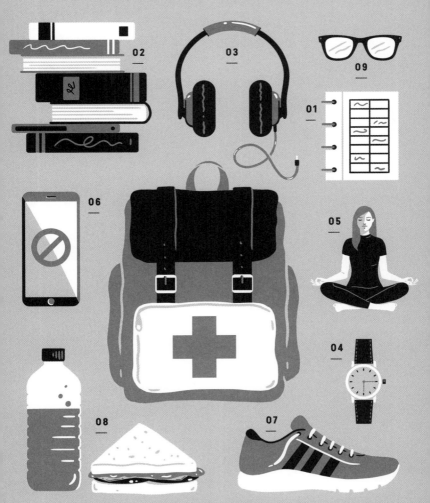

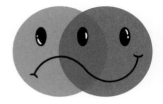

How mood affects concentration

Which came first: how you feel or the mood you're in? Does how you feel affect your mood or does your mood affect how you feel? Either way, there's no doubt that your mood can affect you, and your ability to concentrate.

Moods

Moods are an internal measure of how we are. In psychological terms, a mood is an emotional state but, in contrast to emotions and feelings, moods are less specific, less intense and less likely to be provoked by something that's happened to us. Happy, sad, confident, bewildered, tetchy, calm – we don't express our moods directly but in the way we think, communicate, behave and see the world. Rapidly changing moods can be described as 'mood swings', but generally moods tend to be experienced as positive or negative, and can colour how we feel. If they are particularly overwhelming they can become a form of internal distraction, for better or worse, and disturb our ability to concentrate.

Concentration takes a certain amount of energy and, when we're feeling upbeat and positive, that energy is more readily available. Although concentration may look relaxed on the outside, it is easier if you are feeling positive purely because you have more energy. Moods can fluctuate, and to manage and improve them it's useful to understand what can influence them. It's very difficult to concentrate well when you feel anxious (page 60), for example, as your brain is preoccupied with managing those feelings. Depression (page 61), too, can affect concentration and, if either of these two states of mind become critical, medical help may be necessary. For most of us, however, managing our moods (page 62) can be an effective way to help improve concentration.

Negative thinking

Aligned to mood, it's all too easy to get into patterns of negative thinking, which can create an internal distraction when our thoughts get stuck on repeat. The premise of cognitive behavioural therapy (CBT) is that if we change our thoughts (cognition), this will have an effect on our behaviour, by becoming more positive.

Negative thinking is also very distracting; you're so busy telling yourself you cannot possibly do this job, finish reading that report, prepare a good presentation for your work colleagues that you use up all your energy convincing yourself the task is a lost cause – even before you've started. The upshot? You've no energy left for concentrating on doing a good job. Switch from negative to positive thinking and see how much better you are able to concentrate on what you need or want to accomplish.

Challenging negative thinking takes practice. It helps to be aware of how it can present itself, so if you can identify patterns of negative thinking, you can address it. Look out for these pitfalls and challenge them:

> **All-or-nothing thinking:** Either you're a complete success or a total failure. This thinking can lead to crippling perfectionism.
> **Emotional reasoning:** Believing that you are your mood, i.e. you feel stupid so you must be stupid. This can lead to ...
> **Labelling:** You are stupid! (Again, not true.) Challenge this voice in your head.
> **Overgeneralisation:** If something negative happens, then it must always be going to happen.

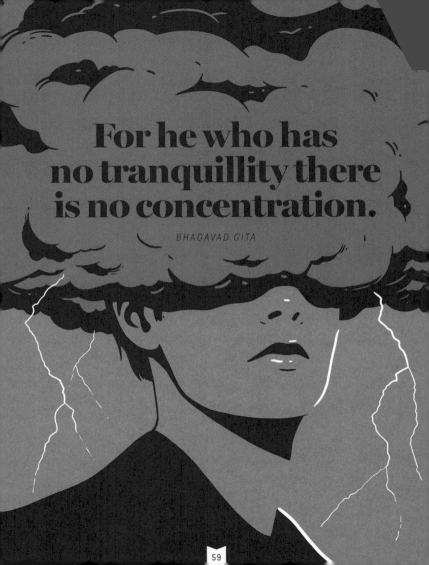

For he who has
no tranquillity there
is no concentration.

BHAGAVAD GITA

> **'Shoulds' and 'musts':** Telling yourself you *should* have done this, or you *must* have done that.
> **Personalisation:** Assuming responsibility, particularly for things outside your control.
> **Negative filter:** Automatically dwelling on the downside and seeing the world in a negative way.

Anxiety

Concentration is severely compromised when we're anxious, and lack of concentration is also a symptom of anxiety. It's easy to see why, because when we are anxious – whether it's about something specific or some insidious and perpetual feeling of unease – we tend to feel physically jittery and unsettled, as if we've OD'd on caffeine. That's the stress hormones adrenaline and cortisol kicking in and, as well as the worrying, this can create the feeling of being constantly on edge, restless and irritable. The physical impact can include muscular tension, headaches, insomnia and early morning waking. It takes a lot of time and energy to manage anxiety, which is itself counterproductive to being able to focus and concentrate for any decent length of time.

If low-grade anxiety continues to escalate it can reach a point comparable to fear, when the freeze/flight/fight response kicks in. This response comes from deep within the more primitive part of the brain, the amygdala, and dates back to more life-threatening times, when a fast response to a sabre-toothed tiger was necessary to survive. If we hit this spot, with its constant surge of stress hormones, even without the tiger, our survival is prioritised

Worry pulls tomorrow's cloud over today's sunshine.

ANON

over our need to think calmly and rationally (that can wait until we're safe again) so the thinking part of our brain – the cognitive frontal cortex that's most capable of concentration – is temporarily annexed.

The freeze/flight/fight response is all well and good when we really are in a life and death situation, but not when our anxiety thermostat is constantly set to 'high' and it inhibits our concentration. Stressed individuals will always struggle with this, so it's worth looking at how low-grade or episodic anxiety can erode our concentration and aggravate the problem.

It's as well to be alert to this as anxiety is an increasing problem, and well worth addressing before it escalates further into a full-blown anxiety or panic disorder or depression. Take immediate steps to rebalance things: reduce distractions, eat nutritiously, exercise, practise meditation, improve sleep – all of which are covered in this book – and seek professional help if it becomes even close to unmanageable.

If you want to conquer the anxiety of life, live in the moment, live in the breath. *Amit Ray, Indian author and spiritual master*

Depression

It's not uncommon to experience depression as a consequence of an anxious state, but it can also be a response to other circumstances or, sometimes, appear to come from nowhere. Poor concentration can sometimes be a symptom of depression. A low level of the neurotransmitter dopamine, often found in those suffering bouts of depression, affects neuro-connectivity and contributes to poor concentration.

Understandably, too, if you are preoccupied by negative or anxious thoughts, suffer poor sleep, lose your appetite and experience feelings of hopelessness, all of which are symptoms of depression, then your concentration is bound to be affected. Winston Churchill referred to his depression as his 'black dog' and one in four of us will experience it, too.

Sometimes depression is reactive – you have good reason to feel low if a close relative has died, you have been physically unwell or have lost your job. It would be unusual not to feel temporarily depressed following events like these. However, it is the creeping, insidious depressions that come about, often for no immediate or obvious reason, that can be tricky – but not impossible – to handle.

Be aware of the early symptoms, and that these can be aggravated by chronic sleep deprivation, poor eating habits, overwork and lack of exercise, and be aware that low-grade physical exhaustion can precede mental depression. No wonder it has become identified as a curse of the have-it-all, do-it-all generation.

MANAGING MOODS

1. Take note and take action, because mild to moderate depression responds well to various self-help measures we can take to help manage our mood.

2. Up your daily exercise – even just 20 minutes' brisk walking can be beneficial, because it helps elevate levels of feel-good brain chemicals.

3. Make sure you get a daily dose of daylight – 20 minutes' exercise in the daylight can make a big difference.

4. Breathing – consciously breathing deeply and calmly reduces feelings of anxiety.

5. Eat regular, nutritious meals – a seesawing blood sugar level aggravates feelings of anxiety.

6. Take time out from your work routine to relax and clear your brain: if you find this difficult, learn to meditate.

7. Keep regular hours and don't get so chronically overtired that all your stress hormones kick in to keep you going, and then keep you awake when you need to sleep.

8. Supplement with the omega-3 essential fatty acid EPA. A gram a day of pharmaceutical-grade EPA was shown to have an equal therapeutic effect in major depressive disorders to 20 mg a day of Prozac, in a 2008 study published in the *Australian and New Zealand Journal of Psychiatry*.

But if none of this works for you, see your doctor. CBT shows good results, and modern drugs have their place, too. Above all, seek help if you need it.

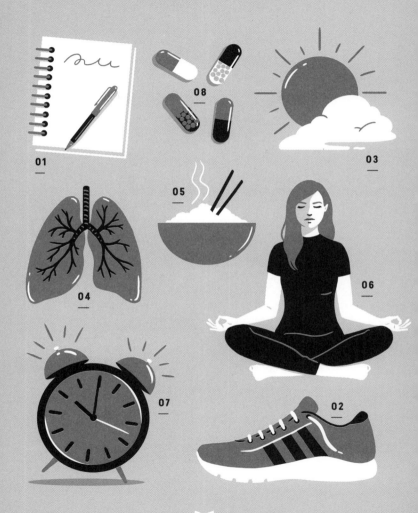

If you're going through hell, keep going.

WINSTON CHURCHILL, BRITISH POLITICIAN

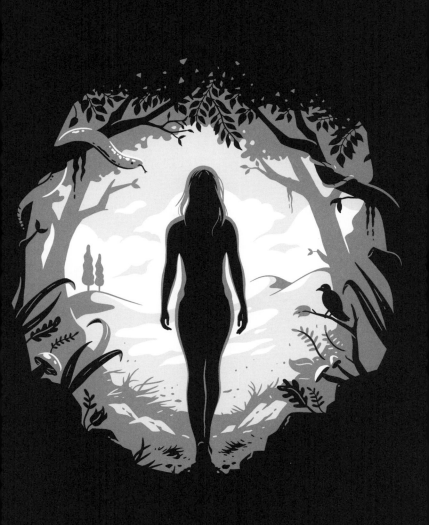

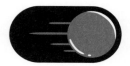

Mindfulness, meditation & the art of switching off

Being able to 'switch off' from distractions is an important part of learning how to concentrate better, for two reasons. One, clearing your mind frees it up to concentrate better, and, secondly, it reduces the general stress of life that can inhibit concentration.

Switching off doesn't come easily to many of us. Learning how to be more mindful, and practising mindfulness or meditation, can all help facilitate greater concentration, not least because feeling calmer as a consequence automatically restores equilibrium and focus.

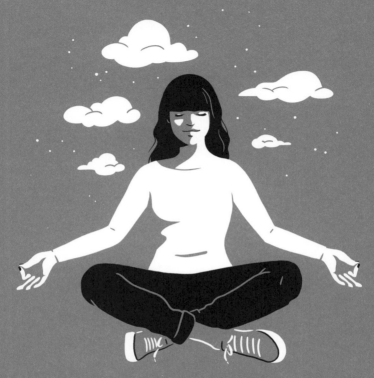

Anyone who knows how to think can meditate.

MAHARISHI MAHESH YOGI, INDIAN GURU

Using the breath

Although we do it automatically, breathing is something that we can also consciously control, making it one of the simplest methods of regaining physical and mental focus and an aid to concentration. Plus it's the single most easily available and useful tool we have for stress management, making it a worthwhile practice for that reason, too.

Feelings come and go like clouds in a windy sky. Conscious breathing is my anchor.

Thich Nhat Hanh, Vietnamese monk, poet and peace activist

Most of us breathe poorly: we tend to over-breathe, taking three or four breaths using only the upper part of our lung capacity, when one good breath using the lungs more completely would serve us better. This shallow breathing is very tiring, not only because we expend unnecessary muscular energy to do so, but because we reduce our oxygen intake per breath. In its extreme form, over-breathing becomes hyperventilation, which can predispose to panic attacks in those who are susceptible.

Meditation is a little drop of perfume that suffuses the day with its grace.

R. D. Laing, psychiatrist

Meditation practice

In all mindfulness or meditation practice, the breath is key. Learning good breathing techniques first will help facilitate this. A daily practice, starting with 10 minutes and building on it, means that the ability to take some restorative 'time out' will also be available to you.

AND BREATHE ...

- Lie comfortably on the floor, knees bent, chin tucked in – what Alexander Technique teachers call the 'constructive rest position' – or sit upright in a chair, legs uncrossed, feet flat on the floor.
- Consciously relax your neck and drop your shoulders, rest your arms by your sides with your palms turned upwards.
- Breathe long and gently through your nose, into your belly, until you see it gently rise, for a slow count of 5.
- Pause, and hold that breath for a count of 5, then gently exhale through your mouth for another count of 5.
- While doing this, try to clear your mind of all other thoughts or, if this is difficult, close your eyes and visualise a pebble dropping into a pool of water and gently sinking down.
- Repeat this breathing cycle 10 times; then see how your regular breathing adjusts.
- You can also use this breathing technique at any time you feel tense or stressed, or as the basis of any meditation practice.

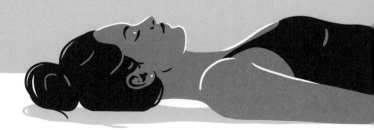

Posture
Bear in mind that poor posture always cramps our breathing, while tension in the muscle with which we breathe, the diaphragm – the sheet of muscle that divides the chest from the abdominal cavity – will also create tension around the aorta, the main artery carrying blood through the centre of our bodies. Tension around the aorta can also elevate blood pressure.

Breathing and exercise
Many physical activities also help improve breathing techniques – singing, swimming, t'ai chi, yoga, walking meditations, playing a musical (wind) instrument, for example. Improving your breathing will immediately improve your overall health and wellbeing, your mental focus and your concentration.

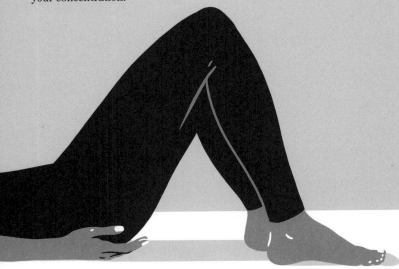

Sleep

Sleep is essential to restore the body and mind. Deep slow-wave sleep, when our brain moves into delta waves, is imperative for proper, restorative sleep – that will restore you physically as well as mentally. Without adequate sleep, not only do we feel tired, irritable, unable to focus or concentrate, it's also a form of physical stress so we produce more stress hormones – adrenaline and cortisol – to compensate, making us even less likely to sleep. Finding it hard to switch on may be because you are finding it hard to switch off.

STAGES OF SLEEP

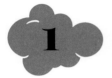

Non-REM sleep is when we move from full wakefulness to the drowsy precursor of sleep, when it's almost inevitable that we will drift off, but not quite. During this phase we are equally capable of either nodding off completely, or waking up instantly.

Is a very definite, but light, sleep cycle and it's during this phase that you might be susceptible to a 'hypnagogic startle', when you are unexpectedly and briefly jolted awake by a muscular jerk. Irritating though this can be, it serves no purpose and does no damage.

Moves you into deeper sleep, where it would be difficult to wake you, although you would respond to a baby's cry, an alarm or other sudden noise or having your name called. Breathing and heart rate are very regular and slow and stable. This is the phase of sleep that restores us physically the most.

Vicious circle

Chronic lack of sleep means that all those 'wake-up' hormones – adrenaline and cortisol – are going into overdrive to compensate for the lack of downtime. Persistent reliance on this state of affairs, rather than taking time off to sleep and properly recuperate, means that your body gets used to feeling wired. Feeling wired begins to feel normal – except you also begin to feel jangled, irritable and less able to concentrate. But it's a vicious circle because, once you've reached this state of hyper-alertness, it becomes harder to switch off.

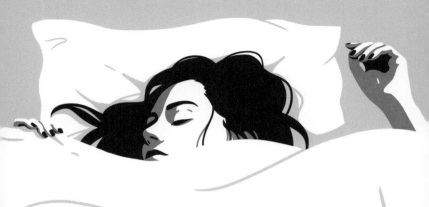

There is a time for many words, and there is also a time for sleep.

HOMER, GREEK POET

Insomnia

Insomnia may be the first obvious sign of a sleep disorder, which further compounds the problem. The more tired you become, conversely the less able you are to relax and sleep soundly. It's important to recognise these early signs of physical adaptation to what is a chronic stress pattern because, in the end, being constantly on 'red alert' begins to affect not only your capacity for concentration, but also your health. In the short term, we cope. In the long term, poor sleep is very stressful physically, and damages our ability to concentrate and function well, affecting everything.

When you're in the throes of insomnia, night waking or inadequate sleep, and suffering all the fatigue of sleep deprivation, it's sometimes hard to know where to start to unravel what the problem is. The good news is that even small changes can make a big difference and you can not only bring about an improvement in how well you sleep, but also enjoy the advantages that good sleep can bring to your ability to concentrate.

EMERGENCY SLEEP TIPS

- Get some fresh air and daylight every day, even if it's for just 20 minutes around the block during your lunch break. Natural light helps to reset your body clock and the natural environment helps relieve stress.
- Factor in some regular, but calming, exercise three times a week – no pumping iron at the gym; opt for walking, yoga, t'ai chi or swimming.
- Eat nutritiously and regularly but cut out caffeinated drinks altogether for the moment – that's tea, coffee and colas – and other artificial stimulants.
- Clear your bedroom of TV, computers, all technology – it should be your calm refuge, designed for sleep: peaceful and dark.
- Keep lights low and just read or listen to soothing music or a calming sleep app before trying to go to sleep.
- Go to bed and get up at a regular hour to help reset your sleep/wake cycle – even at weekends.

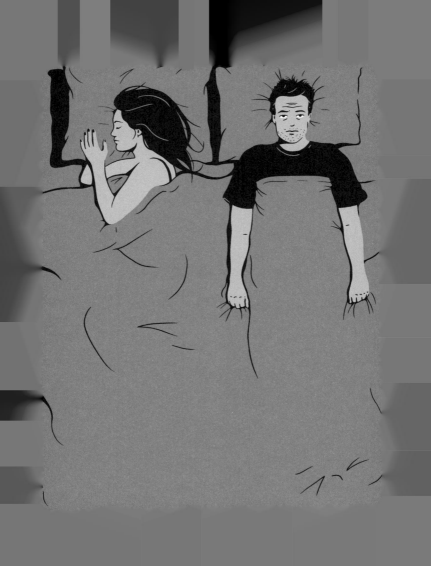

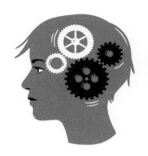

Learning to concentrate

Concentration seems to come more easily to some than to others. Or it may feel as if you have got out of practice somehow, perhaps by constantly trying to multitask, or by allowing distractions to interrupt you. When it doesn't come easily, concentration feels impossible, but this difficulty can be linked to having got out of the habit of it. If it feels as if concentration is very elusive, it might be more possible to manage through the changing of some of our habitual behaviours.

If you do not change direction, you may end up where you are heading. *Lao Tzu, ancient Chinese philosopher and writer*

Habits

Although we often describe habits as 'good' or 'bad', a habit is just a routine of behaviour that becomes a fixed way of thinking about, or doing, something, acquired through repetition. Whether it is a good or bad habit depends on how we feel about it: getting up at 6 a.m. may be a good habit for some, waking at 6 a.m. may be a bad habit for others.

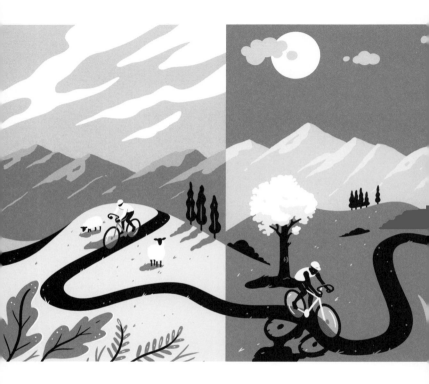

We are what we repeatedly do.

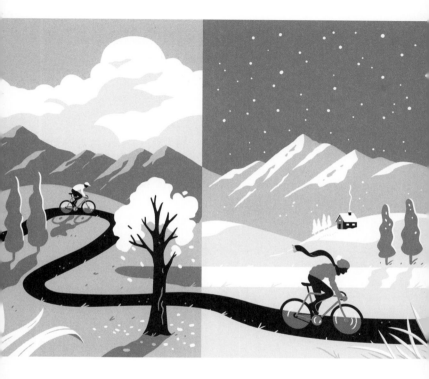

Excellence, then, is not an act, but a habit.

ARISTOTLE, ANCIENT GREEK PHILOSOPHER AND SCIENTIST

Habit accounts for around 43 per cent of our behaviour, according to Wendy Wood, professor of psychology and business studies at the University of Southern California; and those who score highly on self-control, were well motivated and successful at work, did so more through good habit than willpower. 'They automate their behaviours to get them to their goals, so they perform them without even thinking about it.'

It takes time, though, to learn new habits and this we do through self-consciously repeating behaviour until it becomes automatic and, also, reaps its own reward. It takes about three weeks for a repeating behaviour to become a habit, says Jeremy Dean, psychologist and author of *Making Habits, Breaking Habits*. However, there is considerable variation in this and some habits become more automatic more quickly than others.

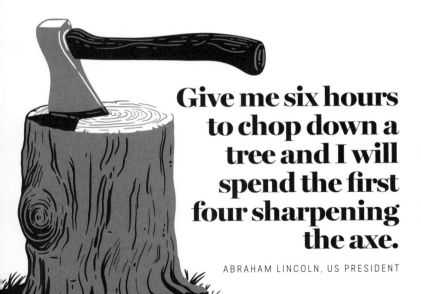

Give me six hours to chop down a tree and I will spend the first four sharpening the axe.

ABRAHAM LINCOLN, US PRESIDENT

Preparation

As concentration is usually in relation to some task, use the working on this to create a physical and mental space to concentrate. This first step, the identification of your personal focus for a definite period of time and without distraction, will make the process of learning to concentrate an easier one. Use a kitchen timer and then forget about the time; consciously put everything out of your mind and practise focusing exclusively on your task.

Engagement

Engagement aids concentration and it takes time to achieve this. There's no point, for example, in only reading for 10 minutes and expecting to reach a better level of concentration. You have to allow yourself time to get into what you're reading, to engage with its content, whether you are reading fiction or a complicated report. The same applies to reaching peak concentration: you need to allow time. Remember that after any interruption, it takes around 15 minutes to reach a good level of concentration again. Eliminate what potential interruptions you can and allow enough time to reach a point of engagement to help enable concentration to become a good habit (page 79).

Motivation

While thinking about how to create habits to support a commitment to concentrating better, it can help personal motivation to think through what factors might be hindering you and those that might help. We all have mind blocks that we are not consciously aware of, so it can be worth shaking these up to help our motivation. Motivation is also helped by reward. Not necessarily in the shape of some sort of chocolate treat, but in the knowledge that it might be possible to get more done, faster and better, rewarding ourselves with more time to do other, more enjoyable things.

Remember, we are 'creatures of habit' and our behavioural habits shape who we are and how we live our lives. So if you want to concentrate better, you first have to make a commitment to wanting to do so and find your motivation. Then take the steps and form those habits that will help you learn to improve your concentration.

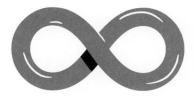

Being in the flow

Professor Mihaly Csikszentmihalyi formulated the concept of 'flow', which he describes as being completely involved and immersed in an activity, for its own sake. When this happens, he explained, ego falls away and time disappears, while every action, movement and thought follows smoothly and inevitably from the one before because the whole of one's being is involved, focused and concentrated on pleasurable engagement with an activity. Sometimes, what we are trying to do is just beyond our ability, so we are stretching our skills and this creates additional focus, all of which contributes to this experience of intense concentration. In this state, what we are trying to accomplish or achieve can seem effortless and without stress.

Athletes refer to it as 'being in the zone', religious mystics as being in 'ecstasy', artists and musicians as 'aesthetic rapture'. Athletes, mystics, and artists all do very different things when they reach flow, yet their descriptions of the experience are remarkably similar.

PROFESSOR MIHALY CSIKSZENTMIHALYI, PSYCHOLOGIST

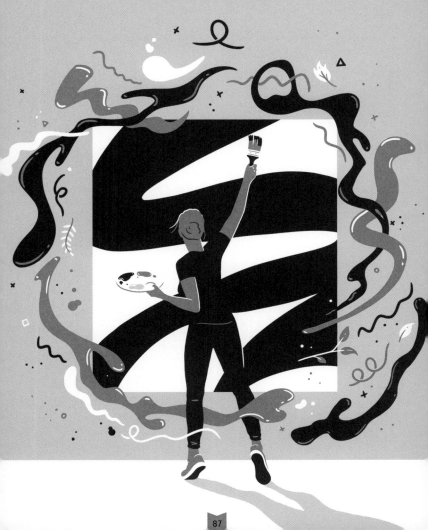

BRAINWAVES

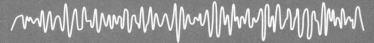

GAMMA WAVES (40–100 Hz): These fastest brainwaves are involved in cognitive functioning, important for memory and learning, and for information processing. Functioning at this capacity over too long a time can be overstimulating and stressful.

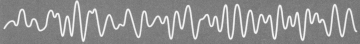

BETA WAVES (12–40 Hz): These occur during normal wakefulness and a heightened state of alertness, enabling us to focus. Again, excessive stimulation of beta waves can be stressful.

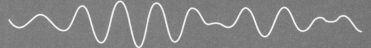

ALPHA WAVES (8–12 Hz): Alpha brainwaves occur when we are focused, daydreaming, very relaxed or during light meditation, which links our conscious and subconscious mind. This is a very creative and 'flow' state of mind.

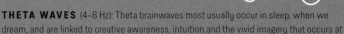

THETA WAVES (4–8 Hz): Theta brainwaves most usually occur in sleep, when we dream, and are linked to creative awareness, intuition and the vivid imagery that occurs at the edge of consciousness.

DELTA WAVES (0–4 Hz): These occur in deep, dreamless sleep and, for some experienced practitioners, during deep, transcendental meditation.

I definitely go into the 'zone' when I play, a mental space no other activity creates. Playing music gives me special insight to everything I do including practising t'ai chi (incorporating rhythm in space and time).

TONY VISCONTI, AMERICAN RECORD PRODUCER AND MUSICIAN

There is a direct correlation between the experience of flow and what happens to our brainwaves and, knowing this, there are ways we can work towards enhancing the positive effects of these by applying what we know to enhance concentration. What's great about the experience of flow is that we can actively feel it when it's happening and learn how to replicate the feeling. Understanding brainwaves and how they need to complement and balance each other is also helpful.

Flow occurs, then, at the border between alpha and theta brainwaves, at that intersection between the conscious and subconscious mind. It can feel almost automatic and comes from a deep confidence, too, in what we are trying to accomplish or achieve. Often this is the result of long practice or application, where we have harnessed our skills to achieve peak concentration or creativity, whether this is physically or mentally.

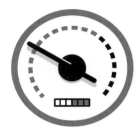

The benefits of slow

You know the feeling. The time between when the alarm clock goes off to the moment you set it again is increasingly a blur. Somehow you get through the day, but by the end of it you can hardly remember what you've done, let alone who you've seen or what you've eaten. Life in the fast lane, it would seem, is running away with you. Trying to do too much, too quickly, in an effort to stay on schedule may be a symptom of 21st century living, but it's beginning to take its toll both emotionally and physically and affects concentration.

The 21st century was destined to be the age of leisure, according to pundits ranging from economist John Maynard Keynes to futurist writer Alvin Toffler, but somehow all that our many labour-saving devices and information technology has done is to raise the stakes. Do more, and do it now – there's no excuse not to get things done in the shortest possible time. There's no need now to ever stop in our 24/7, 365-working-days-a-year society.

No wonder it's difficult to concentrate.

In praise of slow

It was to examine questions like why we continue to live like this, even when we know it's detrimental, that Carl Honoré wrote his book, *In Praise of Slow*. It describes a worldwide movement emerging to challenge the cult of speed. 'The book came about because of a series of articles I wrote about the Slow Movement in the *National Post* (a Canadian newspaper). When I was seriously contemplating the "one-minute bedtime story" to read to my son in an effort to reduce the time it took to read to him I realised it was all too easy to get sucked into the cult of speed. I wanted to find out what others were doing about it.'

Even the search for greater wellbeing can become a tick list, a schedule we have to stay on top of, a tyranny, as we rush from work to the supermarket or after-school clubs. And when we find we are answering emails at 11pm or booking 5am yoga classes to relax, it may be time to reconsider and make better use of our time before it erodes the last remnants of our capacity to concentrate.

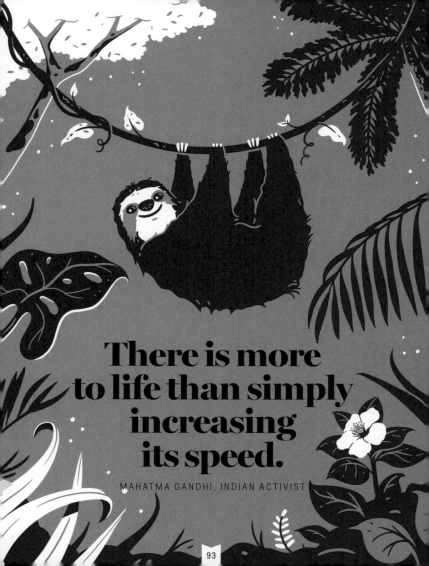

There is more to life than simply increasing its speed.

MAHATMA GANDHI, INDIAN ACTIVIST

EMBRACE THE SLOW: HOW TO DECELERATE

1

Leave holes in the diary rather than striving to fill every moment with activity. Easing the pressure on your time will help you to slow down.

2

Set aside a time of day to turn off all the technology that keeps us buzzing – phones, computers, pagers, email, television, radio. Use the break to sit quietly somewhere, alone with your thoughts. Or try meditation (page 67).

3

Make time for at least one hobby that slows you down, such as reading, painting, gardening or yoga, and use that time to really focus on what you're doing.

4

Eat supper at the table instead of balancing it on your lap in front of the TV and enjoy it, rather than seeing food as mere fuel.

5

Always monitor your speed. If you're doing something more quickly than you need to, simply out of habit, then take a deep breath and slow down.

Time out

The value of taking time out is that it enables the body and mind to reconnect and it reduces the stress that can make concentration so much more difficult. We can take time out in many different ways, through conscious activity to counteract the busyness of daily life, through meditation, sport, exercise or other hobbies, either alone or with friends, which revitalises our engagement with what matters to us.

Times alone are when you can listen to your own mind. That's something we don't allow ourselves today. I was lucky to grow up in that generation before mobile phones. It's fascinating how thought processes today are constantly interrupted. Although we can communicate faster, we are able to think less quickly and less clearly because of these interruptions.

RAY MEARS, BUSHCRAFT EXPERT

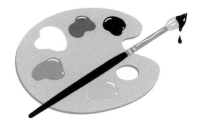

Concentration & creativity

What's the link between concentration and creativity? It may seem initially obvious, insofar as we need to concentrate for long enough for creativity to materialise into something tangible: creative work doesn't just appear, it has to be thought about and worked on to bring it into existence, whether this is a painting or a book. It takes both graft and craft to do this.

Creativity

Creativity is highly prized and sought-after in today's world, demonstrable through entrepreneurial, scientific and even business work, wherever innovation is required. Creative capital can be turned into commercial capital and the trick, as entrepreneur and designer Steve Jobs discovered at Apple, is to work out what people want before they know they want it. This takes creativity, but that, alone, isn't enough. It also takes concentration.

Creativity is just connecting things. When you ask creative people how they did something they feel a little guilty, because they didn't really do it, they just saw something. It seemed obvious to them after a while. That's because they were able to connect experiences they've had and synthesise new things. And the reason they were able to do that was that they've had more experiences or they have thought more about their experiences than other people.

STEVE JOBS, CO-FOUNDER OF APPLE INC.

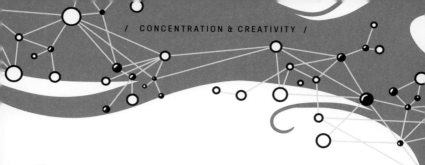

Time

Concentration needs time. Time to explore and engage and learn enough about something in order to build on it: it's just not possible to play the guitar beautifully, learn music or write songs, without the tools – the knowledge of music – you need to do so, and this requires a concentrated effort to reach a point of expertise. The concentration this requires will add greatly to reaping the reward of its outcome. And this applies to anything creative you want to do.

> **It's not that I'm so smart, it's just that I stay with problems longer.**
> *Albert Einstein, theoretical physicist*

Personal creativity is very much the result of an internal process as well as its external manifestation. You can't be creative in a vacuum; it is the result of an interaction between experience, observation and imagination, and these have to be fuelled. The fuelling of ideas requires concentration, too. Thoughts need to be harnessed, sketched, made note of, developed, and then – like a piece of clay – you can begin to mould your ideas into tangible existence. Developing a creative practice will help.

Concentrating on nothing

This may sound like a contradiction in terms. Isn't this just … daydreaming? Procrastination? Time wasting? Not if you are actively concentrating on nothing. This is something advocated by Julia Cameron, author of *The Artist's Way*, and it requires active engagement with the nothing and what comes up. It may feel odd and uncomfortable at first, purely because we are so used to filling every minute of the day with purposeful activity. In a sense you are creating the space to allow the subconscious connections that lie just below the surface of our active minds to shift and connect. Keep a notebook handy!

The act of creativity is also a way to enhance concentration, through the engagement with something that absorbs attention. In the enhancement of concentration, consciously looking for creative opportunities will help this; it's a two-way process – and an enjoyable one, too.

You can't possibly do all your thinking with a consciousness that is constantly distracted. Instead, your unconscious mind is working out problems all the time.

LEONARD M. GIAMBRA, PSYCHOLOGIST

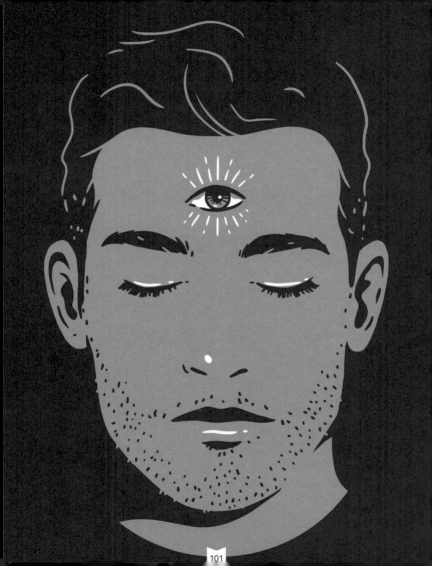

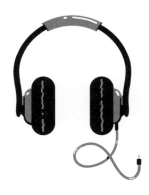

Techniques to practise concentration

Practising concentration is really just about finding things to do that specifically engage you for a period of time to the exclusion of everything else. This will enable you to get a sense of what it actually feels like to concentrate and can help you reach this state of mind more easily through its recognition. What is noticeable, though, is that you can't just go from a state of distraction to one of concentration in 0–60 seconds, in the same way that most of us can't fall asleep the minute our head hits the pillow. It takes a bit of time and, with practice, becomes easier to accomplish.

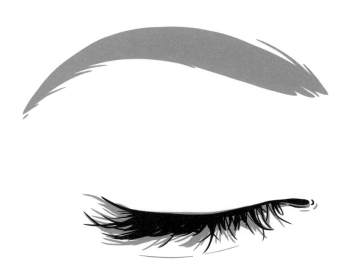

The 'five more' rule

The 'five more' rule is a very simple, but effective, way of learning to concentrate better, and it goes like this: whenever you feel like quitting, just do five more – five more minutes, five more exercises, five more pages – which will extend your focus.

The 'five more' rule is effective because it pushes you just beyond the point of frustration and helps build mental concentration. It's also a form of training as well as being a way of getting something accomplished.

And because the 'five more' rule is a manageable amount, it can be built on and creates its own reward, so it's satisfying and a way of sustaining and extending concentration.

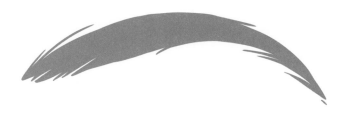

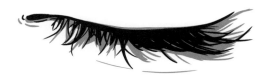

The power to concentrate was the most important thing. Living without this power would be like opening one's eyes without seeing anything.

HARUKI MURAKAMI, JAPANESE AUTHOR

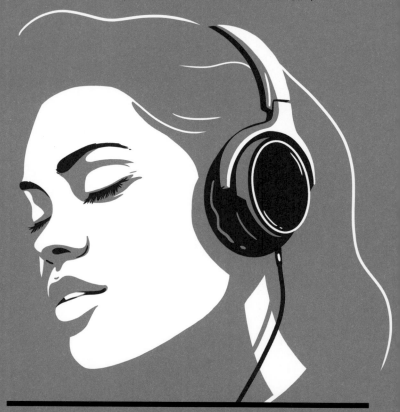

PRESS PAUSE You can utilise timers on your smart phone or other devices to set some 'time out'. There are even apps that can be utilised and one of these is Calm.com, but you can just use a familiar music track to listen to, knowing that it will give you a set amount of time in which to press pause and do nothing.

Sitting still
This is harder than it sounds. It is also akin to meditation (page 67), which can be a useful practice for improving concentration. In this case, however, just get into a comfortable, supported position and sit still and do nothing for five minutes. Use it as a 'pause' between activities, to re-centre. Of course, if you do already practise meditation, combine this with breathing for a restorative 'time out'.

Counting numbers backwards
Counting backwards, in sevens, from 1,000 might sound like an exercise in exasperation, but it does require you to concentrate very hard: try it – 1,000, 993, 986, 979, 972 and so on. It requires persistence and the utilisation of different skills, which for some may include visualising the numbers as they count. Whatever it takes, keep at it for long enough to completely focus, and you'll also have the added bonus of finding that you have temporarily cleared your head of everything else for a few minutes.

Once you've got really good at this, increase the challenge by including a background distraction, something like the radio, just to make the need to focus more intense.

Spelling words backwards
A similar exercise to counting backwards. Start with words that are easy – dog, box, cup – and then build up to longer words, including both nouns and more abstract words – like cushion, blonde, effort, number – increasing the length and complexity of the word, e.g. excessive, radiator or even concentration. Again, this is an exercise that can be built on and extended.

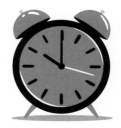

Specific exercises to focus the mind

Many concentration exercises focus on ways to strengthen our attention over a short period of time, because many of us have become so used to only giving something our partial attention (page 38) that this has become a habit. To get back into the habit of concentrating for an extended period of time may need practice, which is the aim of these exercises.

Concentrate: you can't have it all.

Twyla Tharp, American dancer and choreographer

One thing many people who feel they have lost the ability to concentrate mention is that reading a book for pleasure no longer works for them. We have got so used to skim-reading for fast access to information, the demand of a more sophisticated vocabulary, a complex plot structure or a novel's length can make it difficult to engage with. Like anything, single-minded attention may need relearning in order to enjoy reading for pleasure again, but close reading in itself can be a route to better concentration.

Although they don't take long to do, allow enough time to work through a series of exercises every day for several weeks. This will help achieving a good level of concentration to become normalised. It's not necessary to keep to a particular sequence or to do every one every time but, over a period of time, the ability to snap back into concentration should improve and become easier.

Focus

Sit in a comfortable position and find a spot on the wall on which to focus with your eyes. This works best when you have no conscious associations with it to distract you – so, a black spot about 5 cm (2 in) in diameter, at eye level, works well. Focus all your attention on this for around three minutes to start with (you can set a timer if this helps) and let any thoughts that arise drift away, constantly returning your focus to the spot. Anyone familiar with meditation will recognise this technique. If it helps to notice your breath, add this in, but always make your visual focus on the spot your priority. Practised regularly, this can become so familiar it creates a resource on which to draw, enabling you to consciously refocus at will, even without the visual prompt.

To be concentrated means to live fully in the present.
Erich Fromm, psychologist

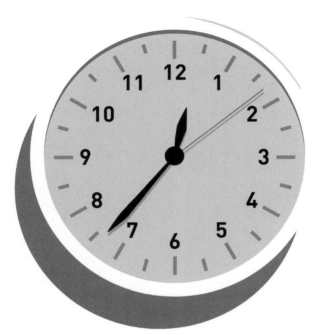

Watching the clock

An old-fashioned clock face with hands and a second hand is needed for this. Starting with the second hand at the 12, focus intently on its progress around the clock face without allowing any distracting thoughts to intervene. Every time your concentration is interrupted by a stray thought, wait until the second hand is at the 12 again, and start over. It's harder than it sounds and can feel very frustrating initially, but give it a go because once the ability is learnt it's easy to access again and again, whenever you need to create a more concentrated state of mind.

Visualisation

We access so much information through what we see, but often we are not particularly observant about what we are looking at, leaving us with just an impression or feeling about what we've seen. In an effort to improve concentration skills, it's worth considering how looking at, and then visualising something can reinforce concentration. Start by paying more attention, whether this is looking at a picture in an art gallery, or taking a bus ride, or just enjoying the scenery from a window. You don't have to commit an exact graphic image to memory, but engage with it, notice details, reflect on it and, within a short time, you will be able to close your eyes and visualise it. There is no right or wrong way to do this; it's just an opportunity to practise focus and improve concentration skills.

Listen attentively

There's a huge difference between hearing and listening. Learning to listen attentively starts quite self-consciously, but will also become a habit that serves you well. You can use music to practise this, the length of a music track giving you between three and five minutes (or longer) on which to focus. Really listen to the nuances of the music, its notes, cadences, instruments used, lyrics. So often music is just a background noise but real, complicated musical notation can be more than just pleasurable, it can be a real boon to helping relearn concentration skills.

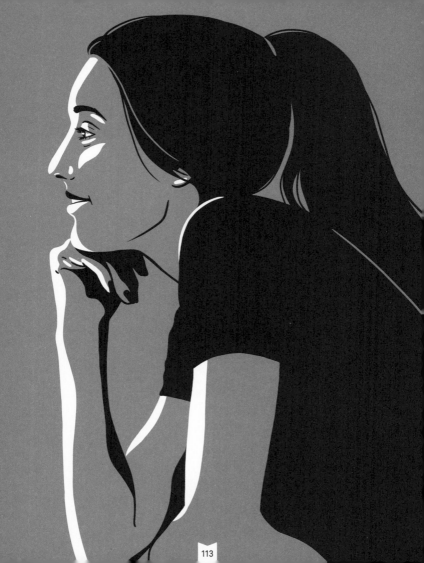

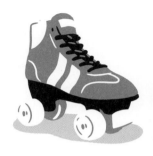

Concentration & memory

Memory is closely linked to concentration, so improving one can help the other. It's also worth considering the way that memory works and the benefit that improved concentration can have on short-term or working memory, and on long-term memory.

Short-term or working memory
We use working memory for things we only need to remember for a short time, for example looking up and then following instructions, like dialling a phone number in the correct sequence. It's the way we hold something in mind and manipulate it, a sort of mental work space, for long enough to use it or follow instructions. Working memory occurs in the prefrontal

cortex of the brain, the area that is involved in more complex executive functions that organise information in a way that we can use it. If we're interrupted before we've completed the task, we will probably have to check the information again because the information is retained for something like 45 seconds, in order to utilise it and then move on. Working memory is used for information we don't need to retain for long, although if repeated numerous times – like a pin number for a bank card – then the information will be transferred from working memory to long-term memory.

Poor working memory *can* be associated with attention deficit hyperactivity disorder (ADHD), but it can also be associated with attention deficit, what we might call a 'poor attention span' or lack of concentration caused by other factors, including stress. Even the physical stress of hunger (low blood sugar) or lack of sleep can have an impact, which is something often seen in young children, although it can apply to us all. So looking at all the ways it's possible to improve concentration skills can really help working memory.

Long-term memory

The process of transferring short-term memory to long-term is called 'consolidation' and this happens over time through a physical process of new, or strengthened, connections developing between the neurons in the brain. This occurs in the hippocampus, located deeper within the brain and closely linked to areas associated with sensory information gained from what we hear or see; and also smell, which is why a particular smell can evoke such a strong memory. There is some evidence to show that the deep stage of sleep is involved in the consolidation of the day's experiences into long-term memory. Once it has been consolidated and committed to long-term memory, being able to recall and retrieve information from long-term memory storage is also important.

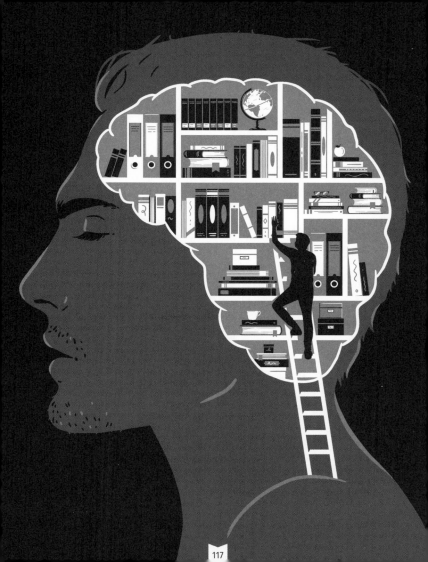

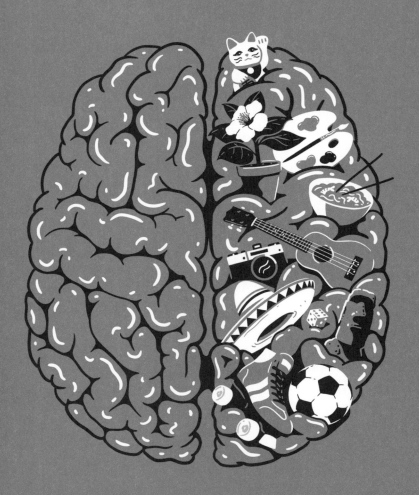

Experience is food for the brain.

BILL WATTERSON, AMERICAN CARTOONIST

Concentration and memory

Some of the activities that we know improve memory, like meditation, also improve concentration. Memory games, like those you may have played as a child, such as Picture Lotto, help concentration too. We have less and less to remember, today, in many ways when our smart phones retain and automatically dial numbers for us, for example. So one way to maintain muscle memory is to exercise it.

One of the reasons why day-to-day memories start to merge into each other is that they become so routine, we don't bother to retain them. So try to vary some of your daily routines. Get off the bus a stop earlier and walk, noticing your surroundings. Make a conscious effort to notice the people around you, identifying something interesting or thought-provoking about them. Choose new foods that you haven't experienced before. Read a book about someone whose lifestyle wouldn't usually appeal. Memorise a poem.

Effect of age?

As we age, our physical senses aren't as acute, but stimulating these helps link different processing systems in the brain. So keep your sense of touch, hearing, taste, smell and sight stimulated by new experiences, or revisiting old ones.

Get into a habit, too, of deliberately creating new memories by remembering and recalling information. Physical exercise (page 121) is proven to help. Create visual links around new information to help consolidate it. Consciously pay attention to and focus on activities and be mindful when you do something, to remember it later so that you are not on the bus to work thinking … did I lock the door?

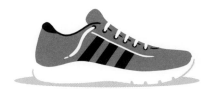

Exercise & concentration

We all know that physical exercise is good for the health of our bodies, but research has shown that it is also good for the brain. Not only does getting physical raise the level of feel-good hormones called endorphins, but it also raises levels of BDNF – brain-derived neurotrophic factor – a sort of 'Miracle-Gro' necessary for cellular regeneration in the brain. 'I cannot overestimate how important regular exercise is in improving the function of the brain,' says John Ratey, Clinical Associate Professor of Psychiatry at Harvard, and author of *Spark! How exercise will improve the performance of your brain*. When we take physical exercise, our working muscles send chemicals into the bloodstream, including a protein known as IGF-1. Once in the brain, this stimulates the production of BDNF, which helps new brain cells, and their connections, to grow.

In addition, levels of other neurotransmitters are increased after the sort of exercise session that will raise your pulse and cause a bit of a sweat for at least 20 minutes. 'Dopamine, serotonin, norepinephrine – all of these are elevated after exercise,' says Ratey. 'So having a workout will help improve focus, help keep you calm and reduce impulsivity.' He goes as far as to describe the effect of exercise as being like a natural dose of Prozac or Ritalin – supporting brain function but without any deleterious side effect.

RATEY'S GOLD STANDARD FOR THE AMOUNT OF EXERCISE WE NEED TO MAKE A DIFFERENCE, WHICH NEEDS TO BE BUILT UP GRADUALLY, IS:

- One hour of moderate exercise (power walking or jogging) four days a week
- A shorter (45-minute burst) of intense activity (squash or running) twice a week
- Combined with strength training and balance drills

And the positive effects continue long after each daily session.

Body and mind

This link between exercise and the mind goes further than just having a direct neurological impact. The actual process of doing something that requires physical expertise, or physical control to coordinate muscles, hit a ball or assume a yoga posture, also requires the sort of exclusive concentration that can, momentarily at least, take your mind off other things. The focus that's necessary, the absence of distraction that occurs when coordinating physical effort, is very helpful in improving concentration.

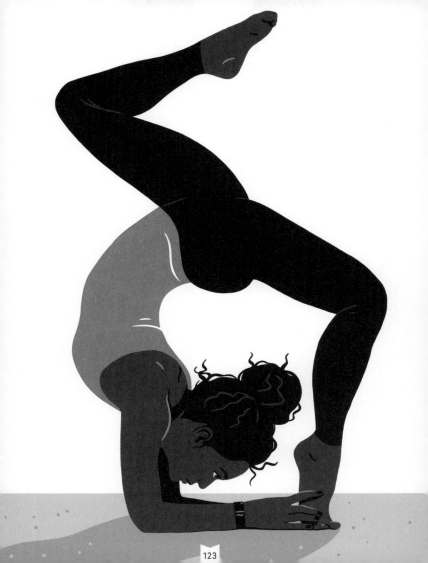

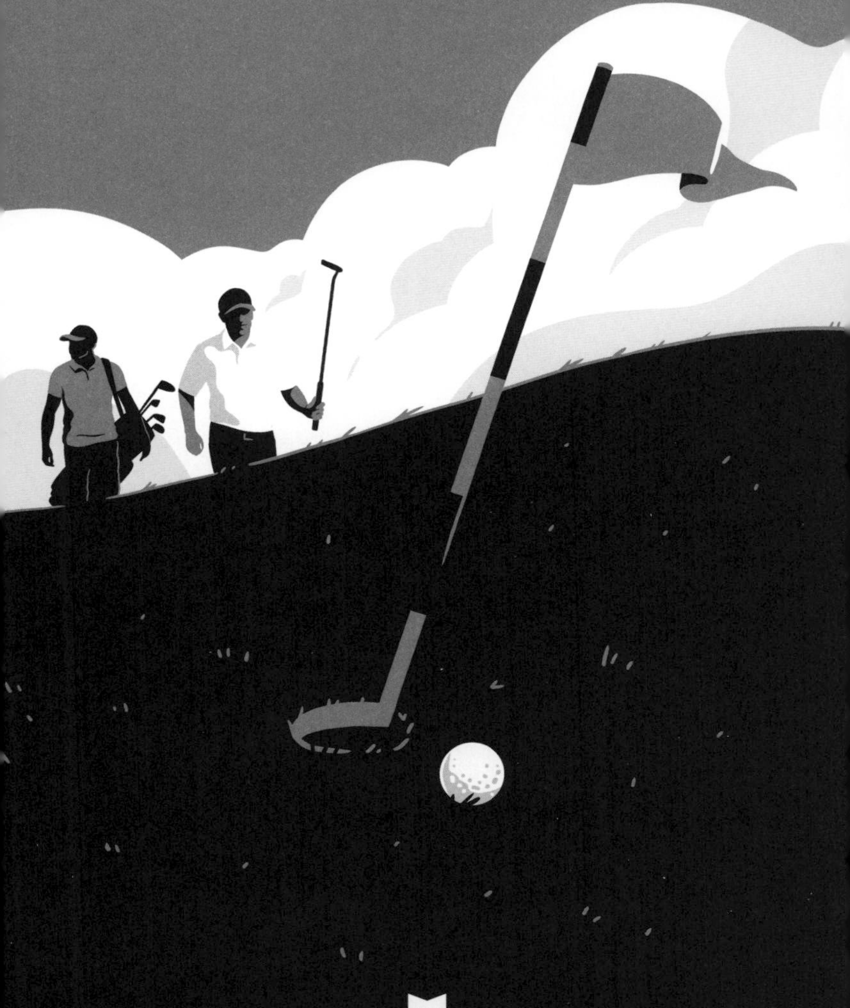

I never hit a shot, not even in practice, without having a very sharp in-focus picture in my head.

JACK NICKLAUS, CHAMPIONSHIP GOLFER

Additional scientific evidence on the benefit of exercise on concentration comes from testing schoolchildren, but it applies to us all, in a Dutch study published in the *Journal of Science and Medicine in Sport* in 2016. It showed that interspersing lessons with a 20-minute stretch of aerobic exercise measurably improved attention spans in the schoolchildren who participated. Another 2014 study from the American Academy of Pediatrics, on the benefits of exercise in seven- to nine-year-olds, not only found that the children's physical health improved as they were fitter, but it also improved their brain function, cognitive performance and their executive control – so not only were the children better able to concentrate but were also less prone to distraction.

Balance

One proviso on the exercise front is not to overdo it. High-intensity workouts, while they can give you an exhilarating exercise high, can also cause physical stress that mirrors the fight/flight response and this can put you in a different zone that temporarily negates cognitive function. This is why exercise can release that cognitive treadmill, but when you want it to aid rather than hinder improvement of concentration, balance is all.

Concentration in everyday life: Checklist

When it comes to concentration, it's not true that you can't teach an old dog new tricks – you can. In fact, learning new tricks helps keep concentration sharp. Recent research has shown that our brains are actually designed to keep active and it's new experiences that will help new brain cells to form throughout our lives, even when we age. Exercising those brain cells regularly – even if it's just by memorising your pin number, your mobile phone number, or even the long number on your credit card – helps foster concentration skills.

New activities
Learning new activities challenges your mental ability just beyond the point of ease and is particularly effective in generating new brain cells (neurogenesis) too. And these new cells will also help energise old brain cells, by firing them up and making new connections, so it's doubly effective. Learning a new language is always cited as a good way to do this, but do it in a way that really engages you. Join a class, for example, rather than listening to a download at home as mutual encouragement can help support your concentration.

Exercise

Physical exercise, for at least 20 minutes a day, when you get slightly out of puff – you could still hold a conversation, but you couldn't sing – has been shown to boost brain power as well as trimming your waist. And if you choose a physical activity that challenges you mentally along with upping your heart rate, you can benefit both at the same time.

Feed your brain

Your brain needs protein, carbohydrates and fats in the right balance, and hydration, so drink lots of water. Oily fish containing essential fatty acids omega-3 – good for your heart, your joints *and* your brain – is recommended twice a week. Always eat breakfast, combining some protein with some carbohydrate, and aim for at least five portions of fruit and veg a day to help make sure you have lots of antioxidants as well as vitamins.

Cut out distractions

If you really want to concentrate, you can. Cut out distractions – turn off the TV, close the door to interruptions – and allow yourself time to really focus. If you are out of the habit of doing one thing at a time, it will feel odd at first. But make the time, and do it until it is done – it doesn't matter whether this is doing the crossword or mastering Photoshop, concentrating deliberately at first will help make concentrating easier in time.

When you write down your ideas you automatically focus your full attention on them. Few if any of us can write one thought and think another at the same time. Thus a pencil and paper make excellent concentration tools.

MICHAEL LEBOEUF,
FORMER PROFESSOR OF MANAGEMENT, UNIVERSITY OF NEW ORLEANS

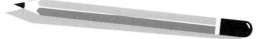

Lists

Making lists is a great way of focusing not just on what you have to do, but prioritising what needs doing first. It also means that once you have written something down and can't forget it, you can put it out of your mind and focus more exclusively on doing the next thing on the list without other things worrying away at the back of your mind and distracting you.

Listen better

We hear with our ears, but we listen with our brains and we are not, generally, very good at what's called 'active listening'. You know what it's like; you ask someone for directions and, because you are distracted by your anxiety about not remembering, or the colour of their hat, you don't really listen. So if you are aware that you're not listening well, actively focus your mind, and engage your brain to receive what's being said – it can really help when it comes to remembering information too, as you are much more likely to retain it if you have really listened.

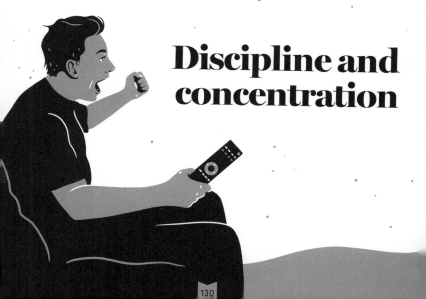

Discipline and concentration

Interest
It's much harder to concentrate on something if it doesn't really interest us. If you have no interest in football, watching a match on TV will probably make little sense to you. However, if you watched it for long enough, or knew a bit about the game's history or the players, it might engage you long enough to hold your attention until it becomes meaningful to you, and you're interested. This process holds with almost anything: stay with it, find out a bit more about it, and see if then you can't connect and enjoy it in a way that enables you to concentrate on it. The same applies to reading a book, assembling flat-pack furniture or learning to waltz.

are a matter of being interested.

TOM KITE, PROFESSIONAL GOLFER

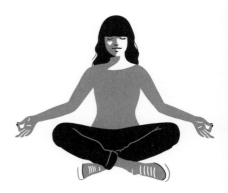

Making the change

How often have you thought, if only I could concentrate better I'd get more done, be less stressed, have greater professional success? And then wondered how to go about improving your ability to concentrate in order to achieve this? When it comes down to it, it's not rocket science and even quite simple steps can make a big difference. What it does take, though, is some commitment to addressing and changing those behaviours that can be counterproductive and reflecting on what is getting in the way of your own personal ability to concentrate.

It's also a question of taking yourself seriously, to believe that you are entitled to create the space and time you need, free from distraction and interruption, for the activities on which you want to focus your precious attention. This can be anything from working on a project that needs to meet a deadline to wanting to spend more time with your children, but whatever the outcome you want, a commitment to its possibility is a first step towards making positive change.

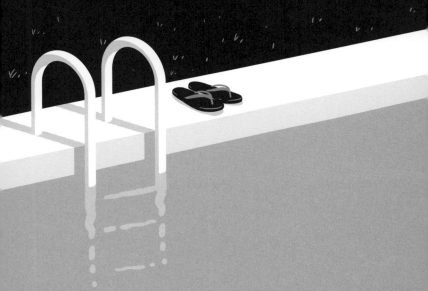

In solitude we give passionate attention to our lives, to our memories, to the details around us.

VIRGINIA WOOLF, AUTHOR

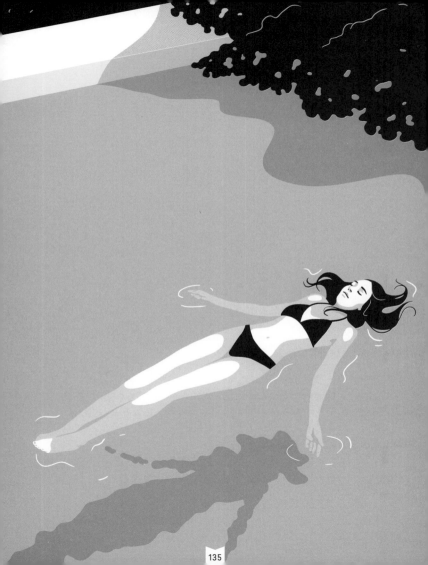

What's also useful is to remember that making changes, while possible, isn't always easy and learning to concentrate better will take time. It's better to make small incremental changes, for example, rather than one sweeping change, which is characteristic of all-or-nothing thinking (page 58), which is known to be difficult to stick with. Generally, we find change quite difficult and if that change means breaking habits of distraction, say, we may well resist it. It's a known fact that, even if their lives depended on it – improving their health after a heart attack, say – only about 20 per cent of people will change their behaviour and embrace its necessity.

This struggle with changing behaviour is partly because it's hard to move out of our comfort zone, out of what feels known and therefore comfortable, into a zone of initial uncertainty. So, for example, the rewards of distraction (a soothing dissociation) can, initially, be experienced more positively than the uncertainty of a quiet, uninterrupted environment and the engagement that allows. The good news is that we are in fact very adaptable and if we have been able to adapt to behaviours that disrupt concentration, then we can re-adapt to those behaviours that foster concentration. Stick with the changes you make until, like all habits (page 79), you are better served by what you're choosing to do and how you're choosing to spend your time.

Insanity is doing the same thing over and over again and expecting different results. *Albert Einstein, theoretical physicist*

The most important thing at this juncture is to know that a) it is possible to change and improve your ability to concentrate; b) making that change will be hugely beneficial to you in the long run; and c) your initial commitment will help motivate you to stick with it until concentrating well whenever you want begins to feel like the new normal for you.

Index

About the author

Harriet Griffey is a journalist, writer and author of numerous books focused on health. Along with *I want to concentrate*, she is the author of six other books in this series: *I want to sleep*, *I want to be calm*, *I want to be organised*, *I want to be confident*, *I want to be happy* and *I want to be creative*, all published by Hardie Grant. Other published books include *Sit Strong* (also published by Hardie Grant), *The Art of Concentration*, *How to Get Pregnant*, and *Give Your Child a Better Start* (with Professor Mike Howe). She originally trained as a nurse and writes and broadcasts regularly on health and health-related issues, is a columnist for *In the Moment* magazine and also an accredited coach with GRIT (www.grit.org.uk)

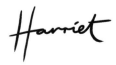

I want to concentrate by Harriet Griffey

First published in 2019 by Hardie Grant Books,
an imprint of Hardie Grant Publishing

Hardie Grant Books (UK)
52–54 Southwark Street
London SE1 1UN

Hardie Grant Books (Australia)
Ground Floor, Building 1
658 Church Street
Melbourne, VIC 3121

hardiegrantbooks.com

British Library Cataloguing-in-Publication Data. A catalogue record
for this book is available from the British Library.

ISBN: 978-1-78488-234-1

Publishing Director: Kate Pollard
Commissioning Editor: Kajal Mistry
Internal and Cover Design: Julia Murray
Internal and Cover Illustrations: Julia Murray
Copy Editor: Kay Delves
Proofreader: Lorraine Jerram
Indexer: Cathy Heath
Colour Reproduction by p2d

Printed and bound in China by Leo Paper Group